Beautifully Made!

Approaching Womanhood
(Book 1)
Second Edition

Edited by
Julie Hiramine

GENERATIONS OF VIRTUE

Contributors:

Julie Hiramine	Mary Whitlock
Sara Raley	Beth Lockhart
Annie Anderson	Chris McCausland
Megan Briggs	Kelsey McCausland

Artwork: Anne Brandenburg
All contributions were made as a free-will gift to Generations of Virtue

Beautifully Made! Approaching Womanhood

Published by: Generations of Virtue
P.O. Box 62253
Colorado Springs, CO 80962
www.generationsofvirtue.org

Printed in the United States of America

ISBN: 978-0-9766143-6-4

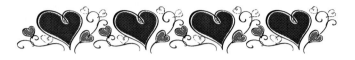

Table of Contents

www.generationsofvirtue.org
"Purity of Heart, Purity of Mind, Purity of Body"

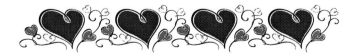

They are all plain to him who understands,
And right to those who find knowledge.

Receive my instruction, and not silver,
And knowledge rather than choice gold;

For wisdom is better than rubies,
And all the things one may desire cannot be
compared with her.

I, wisdom, dwell with prudence,
And find out knowledge and discretion.
Proverbs 8:9-12

Introduction

You have probably been told that you will start your period within the next few years. This is an exciting, wonderful time to learn new things about yourself. This book explains the things that happen before you start your period, what you should do during your period, and other side effects associated with your period. Don't worry, you have nothing to be embarrassed or worried about—your period is a natural event that prepares you for womanhood. When we are talking about your period, all we are referring to is the shedding of the lining in your uterus, which causes blood to come out through your vagina.

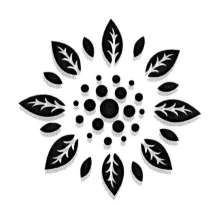

What to Expect in Your Changing Body

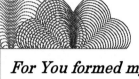

For You formed my inward parts;
You covered me in my mother's
womb. I will praise You, for I am
fearfully and wonderfully made;
Marvelous are Your works, and
that my soul knows very well.
Psalm 139:13-14[1]

Growth Spurt

God designed your body to start becoming a woman at the time that is right for you and no one else. When God tells your body that the time is right, your body starts to release the hormones from your pituitary gland in your brain that will mature you into a woman. One of the first things you might notice is that you are suddenly growing a lot taller. This is normal in girls your age. Some of your friends might also hit what is called a "Growth Spurt."

1. All scriptures are taken from the New King James Version (NKJV) of the Bible.

From the moment God created you in your mom's womb, you have been changing into the woman God designed you to be. Some of those changes were visible and some weren't. At this time in your life you are about to start changing in many ways. You are going to begin changing into the woman God intended you to be. You are growing up! This is an exciting time for you. In this chapter we talk about some of the visible things that you will see in your changing body. These changes that you will see are your body approaching womanhood. After your body is ready, you will begin menstruating. This means that you will start your period.

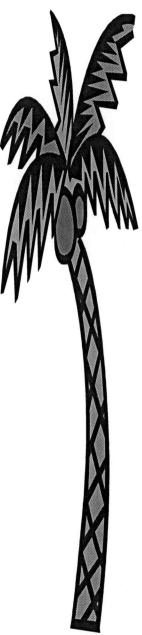

Breasts

One of the most visible changes at this time is that you will begin to grow breasts. This happens with most girls between nine and fourteen, although some girls start earlier and some later. Your breasts will start out small and may be tender and sore at different times while they are grow-ing. Sometimes one breast will grow faster than the other one, but most times they will both be the same size. Some  women have one breast that is bigger than the other, and this is perfectly normal. However God designed your body is perfect for you—you don't have to be like anyone else or look like anyone else.

Hair in New Places

You will also notice that you are getting hair under your arms, in your pubic area (the area between your legs), and on your legs that is darker and more visible. It will be just a few hairs at first, then the hair will become

thicker. Some girls might start to notice hair on their upper lip and a line around their belly button getting darker. Each woman is made differently so no two women will look the same as they go through this time. Some women shave their legs and the area under their arms. Never shave in your pubic area because it will become uncomfortable and itchy and most likely grow back darker and thicker. You can buy shaving gel and a razor to use when you shave your legs and underarms. If you don't have shaving gel, you can use soap just as easily. Make sure you do a good job of lathering the area you are going to shave. If you shave without gel or soap, you could get what is called a razor burn. Using soap or gel protects your skin from the razor while still cutting the hair. Before you shave, ask your mom or someone responsible for you if it is time for you to start shaving.

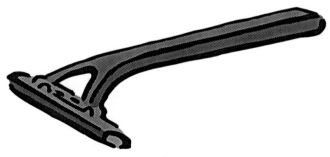

Skin Changes

At this time you might also start getting pimples. This is another sign of hor- mones working in you. The rea- 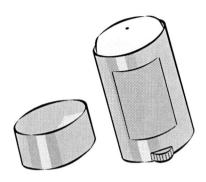 son pimples might pop up where they never have before is that the oil glands in your skin become more active. Your sweat glands will also become more active, which will some- times cause your body to have a more adult odor. Some people use deodorant on their un- derarms to prevent this smell. Showering regularly is one of the best ways to prevent odors.

> **Blessed be the name of God forever and ever, For wisdom and might are His. And He changes the times and the seasons.**
> **Daniel 2:20-21a**

When Will It Happen?

...and all the people rejoiced that God had prepared the people, since the events took place so suddenly.
2 Chronicles 29:36

So you are all ready for your period to start. You might be asking, "When will it happen?" I'm sorry, but there is no way to know when it will happen. You will start your period when God decides it is the time for you, whenever that might be. The best thing you can do is be prepared and know what to do. One gauge of knowing if you should start preparing is if you have developed breasts and have grown more hair. If this has not happened, it is a pretty good guess that you won't start for awhile. You might first notice you have started menstruating when you go to the bathroom and see a little blood on your panties.

Another sign of starting is if you feel a wetness that is not normal. Some girls will have what is called "vaginal discharge" before they start their period; however, this is not your period. Vaginal discharge is a clear liquid that could appear on your panties even before you start your period. Don't be alarmed if this happens. It is another part of your body growing up. What if you start your period while you are not at home? Don't panic! If you aren't in a bathroom, find one and see if it has a dispenser where you can buy a pad.

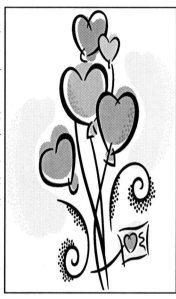

If it doesn't, roll up some toilet paper and put it a little ways up between your legs. If you just lay the toilet paper flat on your panties, it could move around and not stay where it is useful. Lodge it part of the way inside so this does not happen. Then when you get home or somewhere that you can ask someone for a pad, you can change.

15

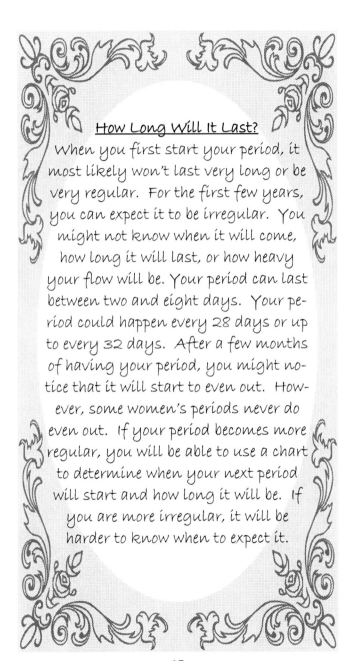

How Long Will It Last?

When you first start your period, it most likely won't last very long or be very regular. For the first few years, you can expect it to be irregular. You might not know when it will come, how long it will last, or how heavy your flow will be. Your period can last between two and eight days. Your period could happen every 28 days or up to every 32 days. After a few months of having your period, you might notice that it will start to even out. However, some women's periods never do even out. If your period becomes more regular, you will be able to use a chart to determine when your next period will start and how long it will be. If you are more irregular, it will be harder to know when to expect it.

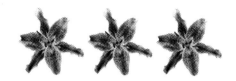

Pads

One of the most common products that women use is the pad. Pads are made of soft cotton and fit in your panties. They have a plastic bottom to prevent leaks and are also sticky on the bottom so they will stay where you put them. Pads come in many shapes and sizes that you can buy according to how heavy or light your flow is when you are on your period. It is usually a good idea to find out which type of pad feels the most comfortable. It might be a good idea to ask your mom which kind she uses, although you might like something different. You may want to try a pad before you start your period so you will know what to do when it does start. Remove the paper backing and stick it on your panties a little towards the front. To dispose of the pad, wrap it in the wrapper that comes with it or in toilet paper and throw it in the trash.

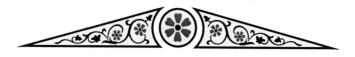

<u>*Never*</u> flush a pad down the toilet. It will get stuck and cause the toilet to overflow, which can be embarrassing besides causing a lot of problems. In most toilet stalls of public rest- rooms there is a trash can of some kind just for the purpose of throwing away these pads. Sometimes pads are a disadvantage, like when you want to go swim- ming. It is not a good idea to go swimming with one on. It would soak up a lot of water and feel un- comfortable.

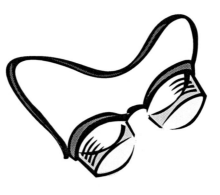

This method is also unsanitary to use in wa- ter because everything on the pad could leak into the water. In the next book you will find out how to use a tampon if you are going to go swimming.

Bra – Why and When You Need One

In like manner also, that the women adorn themselves in modest apparel, with propriety and moderation.
1 Timothy 2:9a

The word *bra* comes from the word *brassiere*. The Merriam Webster 10th Edition Dictionary cites brassiere as: "a woman's undergarment to cover and support the breasts." We wear bras to support our breasts after they become bigger. Breasts are made primarily of fat—there is not much muscle to support them. When we run or do anything strenuous, our breasts can bounce and be uncomfortable. A bra provides us with support to prevent bouncing. We also wear bras to cover our breasts. If you do not wear a bra, your breasts and nipples can move around under your shirt. When you get cold, your nipples can stick out and become more prominent. A bra provides privacy for our breasts.

God created our breasts to nurse our babies when we are older. Our breasts are not to be displayed for others to see.

When Do I Need to Buy a Bra?

You don't need a bra until you start to develop breasts. Before your breasts develop, there is nothing there to support. When you do notice that you are beginning to develop breasts, you can ask your mom or someone close to you to take you shopping for a bra.

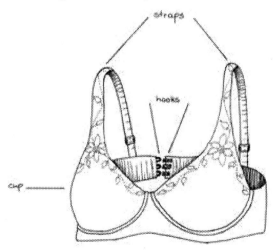

How to Choose a Bra

There are many choices of bras. Comfort is very important in a bra. When you start wearing a bra, you will probably wear it all day, so you will want to choose one that is comfortable to you. For your first bra you probably want to get a fairly simple one and a neutral color (like beige or white) so you can wear it under many different-colored shirts or dresses. There are also many sizes of bras. Your first bra will probably be fairly small because you are just starting to grow. Bras are measured in letters and numbers. The letters represent your cup size and the numbers measure the size around your chest.

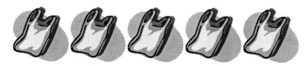

Camisoles

A camisole is a type of undergarment that is worn under a sheer (see-through) blouse or shirt. You could choose to wear a camisole if you would like a little more coverage, even if you don't need to wear a bra yet. Camisoles come in many styles and colors. Again, the same concept applies to buying a camisole as a bra. Buy something that is comfortable and a neutral color.

Biology

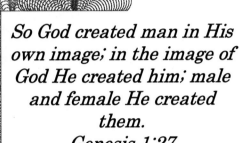

So God created man in His own image; in the image of God He created him; male and female He created them.
Genesis 1:27

When people talk about your period, all they are referring to is the shedding of the lining in your uterus, which causes blood to come out through your vagina. When you start your period, the first thing you will notice is blood in your underwear coming from your vagina. However, there are several things happening inside your body that you will not even notice. In this chapter we address the things that happen inside your body—specifically, in your uterus and ovaries.

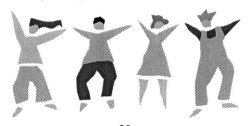

Your period operates in a circle, meaning once it is finished, it starts over again. You have probably heard it called the "menstrual cycle." Your body also releases eggs in a cycle. Do not think that a woman's eggs are like a chicken's eggs; rather, a woman's eggs are microscopic (so small that they're visible only with a microscope) cells.

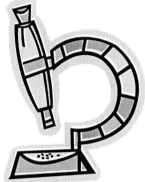

The areas of the body that are primarily involved in your period are the ovaries and the uterus. The ovaries release eggs; the uterus bleeds during your period and is the home to a baby when a woman is pregnant.

When the lining of your uterus starts to shed, you start bleeding, and the blood comes out through your vagina. Don't worry—this is supposed to happen, and it is a necessary function for your body.

After you stop bleeding, the lining of your uterus begins to develop again for the next time you have your period.

Your ovaries release an egg sometime after you're done bleeding. Since the egg is not used, it dissolves.

Isn't it wondrous that God creates our bodies to do something so amazing and complex, yet we don't have to do anything special to make it happen?!

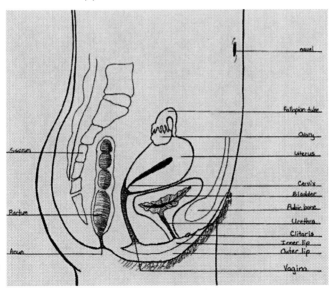

Your Body Image

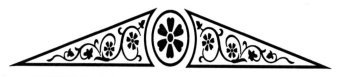

> *For the Lord does not see as man sees; for man looks at the outward appearance, but the Lord looks at the heart.*
> *1 Samuel 16:7b*

Do you ever imagine what you will look like as a grown woman? I sure did. As a child, I would look at myself in the mirror and try to imagine how I might look as a woman. More than anything, I wanted to be beautiful. I would spend long hours daydreaming about the beautiful woman I would be someday. As I grew older, my ideals became slightly more practical, but they didn't change sufficiently. Determined to one day be beautiful, I was very excited to hit puberty. However, I didn't change quite the way I wanted to. In particular, my changing body shape didn't fit the mold of the picture-perfect model image for which I was striving.

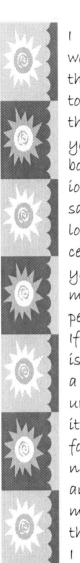

I made the mistake of letting the world's image of the perfect body be the standard I held for my body. In today's culture, this is an easy thing to do. Everywhere you look, you can hardly avoid an impractical body image influencing your opinion about your own body. The message is always the same: "You must look like this if you want to be successful;" "You must have this body if you want people to like you." "You must wear these kinds of clothes so people will look at you." And so on. If you've been led to believe that there is only one way for you to look, it's a lie. There is no one perfect body figure. If there were, we would all have it. I made myself believe these lies for awhile because I thought if I did not, something was wrong with me and I just didn't care enough about my body image. But it was a trap that would only make me miserable. I wasted valuable time trying to reach an unrealistic goal, when all the while God had a much bigger plan for me.

God's plan does not follow the media's agenda. God created us for His perfect plan and His glory. He specifically designed each of us with the body that we need for what He has called us to do. Our body is God's temple, and in order for us to fulfill His purposes, we need to take care of it. Taking care of our bodies is obviously not something the media wants us to do. The media wants us to be obsessed with our physical appearance, especially our weight and our illusion of glamour, whereas God desires us to be focused on our inward beauty. God's wonderful design for you is so much more beautiful than what the world wants you to look like.

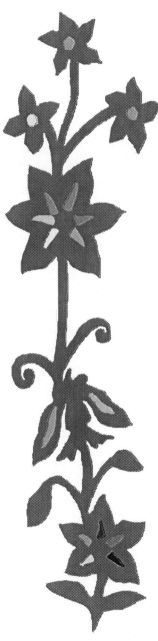

Remember that Jesus loves you more than anyone else does, and He thinks you are absolutely gorgeous.

I still sometimes find myself struggling in this area, but I know now that it is essential to go to the Lord when I'm faced with the pressure to look like something other than what God has intended for me. Be very careful that you don't compare yourself with other people. God made each of us to be unique, and we should be thankful!
-Beth

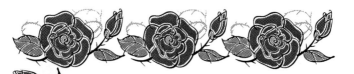

Wrapping Up

Now that you have read these pages together, discuss the following in light of what you have just read:

Do you have any questions for your mom about what your period is and how your body will be changing?

How do you feel about what will be going on inside and outside your body in the future?

Ask your mom about when her period first started and how old she was.

How do you feel about starting to wear a bra?

After reading this, do you feel prepared if your period starts when you are not at home? Do you know what to do?

What are ways you can be thankful about God's wonderful design for your body?

A Word About Generations of Virtue

The ministry of Generations of Virtue believes God is raising this current generation to be godly men and women with pure hearts, minds, and bodies. We long to see our society become one that worships God with its whole being. Our vision is that of a generation that does not look to meaningless, vain relationships for comfort. We long to see a generation that calls to God to be its number one adviser and guardian. This goal, we believe, is to be attained through the help of parents. For this reason, Generations of Virtue provides parents and teens with the counsel and resources they need to discover God's gift of purity and His promise to be the protector of our love lives.

Generations of Virtue does not simply promote abstinence. We believe in the merits of courtship and the importance of emotional, spiritual, and physical purity. If you are looking for resources to teach your children about God's design for romance and relationships, or if you are a teen looking to find the truth about purity, we invite you to take a look at our website and the resources we offer. Generations of Virtue is an up-and-coming organization, so look for new additions as we grow.

www.generationsofvirtue.org

Celebrating Womanhood: Book 2 in the Beautifully Made! Series-

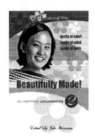

Celebrating Womanhood- Having your period is something to celebrate, and this booklet explains why. The second book in the *Beautifully Made!* series, *Celebrating Womanhood* covers subjects like "PMS", which products to use and how to use them, tips on health, and much more. You and your daughter can share quality mother-daughter time as you read and discuss this book; afterward, she can keep the booklet as a continuous reference. Biblically centered, this book will give your daughter an encouraging message about her period. **Recommended as a gift for your daughter at the start of her first period.**

Wisdom from a Woman:
A Mother's Guide:
Book 3 in the *Beautifully Made!* Series-

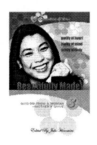

Wisdom from a Woman : A Mother's Guide- Are you anxious about your daughter starting her period? Generations of Virtue has compiled a wonderful resource for mothers to lovingly guide their daughters into womanhood. This book contains ideas on how to celebrate with your daughter, a fabulous section on the biology behind women's bodies, how and when to tell your daughter about her period, and some of the surprises associated with a developing daughter (for instance, mood swings). This biblically-focused book can help every mother explain some of the intricacies of womanhood to her precious girl.

www.generationsofvirtue.org
"Purity of Heart, Purity of Mind, Purity of Body"

AVAILABLE FOR THE FIRST TIME ON AUDIO CD!

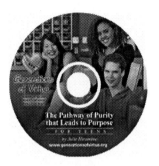

The Pathway of Purity that Leads to Purpose
by Julie Hiramine

Using the 5 senses of seeing, feeling, tasting, hearing, and smelling, Julie Hiramine will not be your science instructor, but edifying you in order to stay pure. In today's world, there is a flood of inappropriate imagery and explicit content that besieges us everywhere we turn. God's call on this generation is to step up into His higher standard and seek His face in the midst of all that wants to pull us off course. Teens need to learn how to navigate through the maze the world is currently lost in with their eyes on Jesus as their guide. Teens will receive practical guidance on how to meet the many challenges that surround them in the areas of dating versus courtship, media discernment, and developing a deeper relationship with the Lord in this captivating presentation. **Recommended for teens and parents.**

If you enjoyed this resource, please order these other recommended resources found on our website.

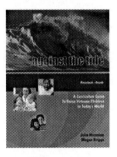

Against the Tide Elementary Guide

By
Julie Hiramine and Megan Briggs

Age-appropriate training for young ones!

God calls His people to be set apart from the world; He calls us to be sanctified. In an effort to accomplish this requirement, Julie Hiramine and Megan Briggs have organized a curriculum guide for the preschool to fourth grade years designed to train your children in purity and to solidify the process of character development. *Against the Tide— Elementary* is a year-by-year guide covering the basics of where babies come from, modesty, manners, and character development through assignments from resources Generations of Virtue feels are beneficial for young children. This guide focuses on building a solid foundation for the road to adulthood with age-appropriate character building and sex education.

Against the Tide Middle School Guide

By
Julie Hiramine and Megan Briggs

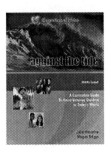

Practical Training for Preteens!

The 'tween years are a pivotal time in the shaping of your child's convictions, body image, relationship with figures of authority, and more. This curriculum guide is for 10- to 14-year olds and, like its predecessor for elementary-aged children, highlights when and how to use age-appropriate sex education and character training. *Against the Tide—Middle School* will help parents and children establish a practical approach to purity training. After reviewing hundreds of products, this guide will take you through the resources we have found to be most beneficial for young people. Also included with this guide are free updates every year in order to keep you posted on the new, up-to-date resources we have found after a year of searching. Take the leg-work out of establishing a purity-training plan with this excellent guide.

Printed in the United States
99255LV00003B/391-486/A

9 780976 614364